"The Psychology of Weight Loss: Rewiring Your Mind for Long-Term Success"

Introduction: The Hidden Key to Weight Loss

Overview: Why weight loss isn't just a physical challenge but a mental and emotional one. The concept of rewiring thought patterns, overcoming self-sabotage, and developing a mindset that supports long-term success.

Chapters

Chapter 1: Understanding Your Weight Loss Mindset

Exploring how beliefs, past experiences, and societal conditioning shape one's approach to weight loss & the concept of limiting beliefs and self-sabotage.

- What is a mindset?

- Identifying negative thought patterns.

- The power of self-awareness.

Exercises:

- Write down three beliefs about weight loss and analyze their origins.

- Journal daily to uncover recurring thoughts about food and body image.

Chapter 2: The Role of Emotional Eating

Examining how emotions influence eating habits and lead to overeating & how food becomes a coping mechanism and the triggers behind emotional eating.

- Emotional hunger vs. physical hunger.

- Common triggers for emotional eating.

- Breaking the reward-punishment cycle.

Exercises:

- Keep an emotion-food diary for one week.

- Practice the HALT technique (Ask: Am I Hungry, Angry, Lonely, or Tired?).

Chapter 3: Overcoming Self-Sabotage

Analyzing the subconscious behaviours that derail progress, such as fear of failure, perfectionism, or using food as comfort.

- Recognizing self-sabotage patterns.

- Understanding the role of fear and resistance.

- Building self-compassion.

Exercises:

- List examples of self-sabotage and reframe each with a positive alternative.

- Create a self-compassion mantra to use during setbacks.

Chapter 4: Rewiring Negative Body Image

Explore how body image impacts self-esteem and weight loss efforts & how to cultivate body positivity and acceptance as a foundation for change.

- The link between body image and self-worth.

- Media and societal pressures.

- Practicing self-acceptance while striving for improvement.

Exercises:

- Stand in front of a mirror daily and name three things you appreciate about your body.

- Create a "body gratitude" journal.

Chapter 5: The Science of Habits and Weight Loss

Dive into how habits are formed and how to replace destructive habits with positive ones. Introduce habit-stacking and other behavioural strategies.

- The habit loop: cue, routine, reward.

- Breaking bad habits without guilt.

- The power of small, consistent actions.

Exercises:

- Identify one "trigger" and design a healthier response.

- Start one new positive habit using the two-minute rule.

Chapter 6: Managing Stress Without Derailing Your Goals

How chronic stress disrupt weight loss efforts by affecting hormones, cravings, and mental clarity.

- Cortisol and its impact on weight.

- Managing stress through mindfulness.

Exercises:

- Practice 5 minutes of mindfulness meditation daily.

Chapter 7: Building Resilience and Motivation

How to handle setbacks and stay motivated during the weight loss journey. Focus on resilience as a skill that can be developed.

- The myth of willpower vs. discipline

- Strategies for staying motivated long-term.

- Reframing failure as a learning opportunity.

Exercises:

- Write down three past setbacks and what you learned from them.

- Set a monthly reward system for non-scale victories.

Chapter 8: The Power of Self-Compassion in Weight Loss

Self-compassion is the antidote to this destructive pattern. It's about being kind and understanding toward yourself, especially when things don't go as planned.

- What Is Self-Compassion?
- Self-Criticism Hurts More Than It Helps
- The Impact of Self-Compassion on Long-Term Weight Loss

Exercises:

- The Garden Analogy
- The Coach Analogy
- The Slippery Slope Analogy

Chapter 9: Visualizing Success and Setting Goals

Explore the power of discovering your true motivation—the deeper *why* that fuels your weight loss journey. When your motivation is rooted in a sense of purpose, it becomes the driving force that helps you overcome challenges, stay consistent, and create lasting change in your life.

- Motivation Beyond the Surface
- Connecting to Your Deeper Purpose
- Your "Why" Provides Consistency

Exercises:
- Write Down Your "Why"
- Create a Vision Board
- Dig Deeper with the "5 Whys"

Chapter 10: Celebrating Progress and Building Long-Term Success

Celebrating progress is essential for maintaining motivation, boosting self-confidence, and building a foundation for long-term success. By acknowledging your wins—no matter how small—you shift your mindset from one of scarcity and frustration to one of abundance and achievement.

- Progress Is Built on Consistency, Not Perfection
- Celebrating Boosts Motivation and Reinforces Positive Behaviours.
- The Role of Self-Compassion in Celebration

Exercises:
- Keep a "Win Journal"
- Set Micro-Goals and Reward Yourself
- Your Successes with Others
- Share

- Create Non-Food Rewards
- Reflect on Your Journey Regularly

Conclusion: Embracing the Journey

Chapter 1: Understanding Your Weight Loss Mindset

Introduction: The Invisible Roadblock

Imagine preparing for a long road trip, but your GPS is set to the wrong destination. No matter how hard you drive, you'll never get where you want to go. This is what happens when you approach weight loss with a mindset that's working against you.

Most people believe weight loss is simply about eating less and exercising more, but the truth is, your thoughts, beliefs, and emotions shape every decision you make. This chapter will help you uncover the invisible roadblocks in your mind and begin to reset your "mental GPS" for long-term success.

Shaping Your Mindset

1. The Role of Beliefs
Your mindset is a collection of beliefs formed by experiences, culture, and societal messages. For example, if you've ever thought, *"I'll never lose weight because I don't have enough willpower,"* that's a limiting belief. These beliefs act like invisible chains, holding you back from taking action or staying consistent.

Studies show that people who believe weight loss is out of their control are less likely to succeed, even when provided with the right tools. Changing this belief increases the likelihood of success.

2. The Power of Self-Talk
The way you talk to yourself influences your actions. Negative self-talk like, *"I'm so bad for eating that cake,"* creates guilt, which can lead to emotional eating or giving up altogether. Positive self-talk, on the other hand, fosters resilience.

Imagine two people miss a workout. One says, *"I'm such a failure; I can't stick to anything."* The other says, *"One missed workout doesn't define me. I'll get back on track tomorrow."* Guess who stays consistent?

3. The Influence of Past Experiences

Your weight loss mindset is often shaped by past attempts. If you've failed before, you might approach new efforts with skepticism, thinking, *"Why bother? I'll just fail again."* This creates a self-fulfilling prophecy.

Someone who's experienced restrictive dieting may associate weight loss with misery, making it harder to embrace balanced approaches.

Practical Strategies for Immediate Use

1. **Identify Limiting Beliefs**
Write down three beliefs you have about weight loss (e.g., "I don't have enough time to exercise"). Challenge each one by asking: *Is this true? What evidence do I have?* Replace them with empowering beliefs (e.g., "I can find 10 minutes a day to move my body").

2. **Practice Positive Self-Talk**
Replace harsh inner dialogue with supportive phrases. For example, instead of saying, *"I can't resist junk food,"* try, *"I'm learning to make healthier choices."*

3. **Rewrite Your Story**
Reflect on past weight loss attempts and identify what went wrong. Instead of seeing them as failures, frame them as learning experiences. Ask yourself: *What did I learn about myself? How can I do better this time?*

Simplifying the Ideas

1. **Beliefs as Filters**:
Imagine wearing sunglasses with a dark tint. The world isn't actually darker, but your perception is. Limiting beliefs act like these sunglasses, distorting how you see challenges and opportunities. Replacing them is like switching to clear lenses—you'll see things as they truly are.

2. **Self-Talk as a Coach**:
Picture your inner voice as a coach on the sidelines. A critical coach shouting, *"You're terrible at this!"* won't motivate you. But a coach saying, *"You've got this—keep going!"* pushes you forward. Become your own encouraging coach.

Summary:

- **Your mindset matters**: Weight loss begins in your mind, not your plate.
- **Beliefs influence behaviour**: Identifying and challenging limiting beliefs is crucial.
- **Self-talk shapes outcomes**: Be kind and supportive to yourself for better results.
- **Your past is a teacher**: Use lessons from previous attempts to build a better approach.

Next Chapter: The Role of Emotional Eating

Now that you understand how mindset shapes your weight loss journey, it's time to address one of the biggest roadblocks: emotional eating. In the next chapter, we'll uncover why emotions often drive food choices and how to break the cycle for good.

This chapter lays a strong foundation by blending self-awareness with actionable strategies, motivating you to take ownership of your mindset and move forward with confidence.

Chapter 2: The Role of Emotional Eating

Introduction: When Hunger Isn't About Food

Have you ever found yourself reaching for a bag of chips after a stressful day, or eating ice cream not because you're hungry, but because you're feeling lonely? This is emotional eating—a habit that ties your feelings to food, often without you even realizing it.

Emotional eating is one of the biggest obstacles to weight loss. It creates a cycle where food becomes a way to numb emotions instead of fuel for your body. In this chapter, we'll explore why emotions drive food choices, how to identify your triggers, and practical ways to break free from the cycle.

Understanding Emotional Eating

1. Emotional Hunger vs. Physical Hunger
Emotional hunger often strikes suddenly and feels urgent, while physical hunger develops gradually and can be satisfied by almost any food. Emotional hunger craves specific comfort foods, like sweets or carbs, and tends to leave you feeling guilty afterward.

A 2020 study found that 40% of people report overeating or eating unhealthy foods in response to stress. Understanding this difference is the first step to breaking the habit.

2. Common Emotional Triggers
Emotional eating is often triggered by negative feelings like stress, boredom, loneliness, or sadness, but it can also stem from positive emotions, such as celebrating with food.

- Stress: Grabbing fast food after a long day at work.

- Boredom: Mindlessly snacking while watching TV.

- Happiness: Overindulging at a party to "reward yourself."

3. The Cycle of Emotional Eating
The cycle starts with a trigger (stress or boredom), followed by eating for comfort, which provides a temporary relief. But this is often followed by guilt or frustration, leading to more emotional triggers—and the cycle repeats.

Think of someone who feels stressed at work. They eat a donut for comfort, feel guilty about it later, and then eat more to suppress that guilt.

Tips:

1. Identify Your Triggers

Keep a food-mood journal to track what you eat and how you feel before and after. Patterns will emerge that reveal your emotional eating triggers.

2. Develop a "Pause Plan"

When you feel the urge to eat, pause and ask yourself: *Am I physically hungry?* If the answer is no, identify what you're feeling instead (e.g., stressed, bored).

3. Find Non-Food Coping Mechanisms

- Replace emotional eating with activities that provide comfort without calories:

- Stress: Take a walk or practice deep breathing.

- Boredom: Try a hobby like drawing or reading.

- Sadness: Call a supportive friend or journal your thoughts.

4. Practice Mindful Eating

- When you do eat, focus entirely on the experience. Sit down, chew slowly, and savor each bite. This helps you stay   connected to your body's hunger and fullness signals.

Simplifying the Ideas

1. **Filling a Leak with Food**:
Emotional eating is like trying to fill a leaking bucket with water. No matter how much you pour in, the leak (your emotions) remains unless you address the source of the problem.

2.   **The Emotional Thermostat**:
Imagine your emotions as a thermostat. Emotional eating is like temporarily raising the heat when you're cold, but not fixing the broken furnace that's

causing the chill. To truly stay warm, you need to fix the furnace—your
underlying feelings.

Key Takeaways

- **Emotional hunger vs. physical hunger**: Learn to recognize the difference.

- **Triggers matter**: Identify emotional eating triggers through awareness and
journaling.

- **Break the cycle**: Replace food with healthier coping mechanisms.

- **Mindfulness is key**: Staying present while eating helps prevent overeating.

Preview of Next Chapter: Overcoming Self-Sabotage

Now that you understand how emotions influence your eating habits, we'll turn
to another common roadblock: self-sabotage. In the next chapter, we'll explore
why you might unconsciously derail your own progress and how to stop this
pattern for good.

This chapter engages readers by shedding light on an experience many struggle
with, while empowering them with clear strategies to regain control.

Chapter 3: Overcoming Self-Sabotage

Introduction: The Enemy Within

Picture this: you're on track with your weight loss journey, eating balanced
meals, staying active, and feeling good about your progress. Then, out of
nowhere, you skip a workout, binge on junk food, or tell yourself, *"I'll start again
on Monday."* Sound familiar?

This is self-sabotage—a pattern of behaviors or thoughts that undermine your
progress, often driven by fear, doubt, or deeply ingrained habits. In this chapter,
we'll uncover why you might unconsciously work against yourself and how to
break free from these patterns to achieve long-term success.

Understanding Self-Sabotage

1. The Fear of Success or Failure
Self-sabotage often stems from a fear of the unknown. Success might mean
changes in relationships, expectations, or identity, while failure reinforces
negative beliefs about you. Either way, these fears can cause you to stall your
progress.

Someone might fear losing weight because they associate being thinner with receiving unwanted attention. Another person might sabotage themselves because they believe deep down they'll fail, so they avoid trying too hard.

Studies show that 70% of people experience "imposter syndrome" in various areas of life, which can include weight loss—a fear of not being worthy of success.

2. Perfectionism and the "All-or-Nothing" Mentality

The belief that you have to be perfect to succeed is a major driver of self-sabotage. When perfection isn't achieved, people often give up entirely.

Missing one workout leads to abandoning the entire exercise plan, or eating one "unhealthy" meal spirals into a weekend of overeating. Research has shown that perfectionism increases stress and reduces the likelihood of achieving goals.

3. Using Food as a Reward or Punishment

For many, food becomes a tool for self-sabotage, whether by rewarding good behavior or punishing perceived failures. Telling yourself, *"I worked out today, so I deserve dessert,"* can lead to overindulgence. Conversely, thinking, *"I ate badly, so I might as well keep going,"* perpetuates the cycle.

Practical Strategies for Immediate Use

1. Identify Your Sabotage Triggers

- Write down moments when you've sabotaged your progress in the past. Ask yourself: *What was I feeling at the time? What was I afraid of?* Recognizing patterns is the first step to breaking them.

2. Shift from "All-or-Nothing" to "Good-Enough"

- Embrace flexibility. Instead of thinking you need to work out for an hour, aim for 10 minutes. Small steps are still progress.

- Practice self-forgiveness: missing one meal or workout doesn't mean you've failed.

3. Create New Rewards

- Replace food rewards with non-food alternatives that align with your goals. For example:

- Treat yourself to a new workout outfit.

- Celebrate progress with a relaxing activity, like a bubble bath or a movie night.

4. Use Visualization to Overcome Fear

   • Visualize your future self succeeding. Imagine how good it feels to reach your goal. Confront the fear of change by focusing on the positive aspects of your transformation.

5. Build Accountability

   • Share your goals with a trusted friend, coach, or support group. Having someone to check in with can keep you motivated and reduce self-sabotage tendencies.

Simplifying the Ideas

1.   **The Saboteur Within**
Self-sabotage is like having an inner "anti-coach" who whispers doubts and excuses in your ear. To overcome it, you need to recognize its voice and replace it with a supportive inner coach.

2.   **The Perfectionist's Ladder**
Imagine climbing a ladder to success. Perfectionists demand that they climb every rung perfectly. If they slip once, they jump off entirely. A better approach is to hold on, regain balance, and keep climbing.

3.   **The Broken Compass**
Self-sabotage is like using a compass that points in the wrong direction. It may feel like you're making progress, but it leads you away from your goals unless you recalibrate.

Key Takeaways

   • **Fear and perfectionism fuel self-sabotage**: Recognize and confront these patterns.

   • **Flexibility is key**: Small efforts and self-compassion lead to sustained progress.

   • **Food is not a tool for rewards or punishment**: Shift to healthier motivators.

   • **Accountability and visualization help**: Build a strong support system and focus on your goals.

Next Chapter: Rewiring Negative Body Image

Now that you've tackled self-sabotage, it's time to address how you view yourself. In the next chapter, we'll explore the impact of negative body image and teach you how to foster self-acceptance while striving for improvement.

This chapter empowers readers to recognize self-sabotage as a common but conquerable obstacle, leaving them motivated and equipped with tools for personal growth.

Chapter 4: Rewiring Negative Body Image

Introduction: Loving the Mirror Again

How do you feel when you look in the mirror? For many, the answer is far from positive. Negative body image isn't just about appearance—it impacts your self-esteem, mental health, and ability to stay motivated on your weight loss journey.

If you've ever thought, *"I'll only be happy when I reach my goal weight,"* you're not alone. But this mindset traps you in a cycle of self-criticism, making it harder to achieve lasting success. This chapter will teach you how to challenge and rewire negative body image, helping you build self-acceptance while working toward your goals.

Understanding and Reframing Body Image

1. What Is Body Image?

Body image is the mental picture you have of your body and how you feel about it. It's influenced by personal experiences, societal standards, and even family comments. Negative body image distorts this picture, making you overly critical and ashamed of your appearance.

A study by the National Eating Disorders Association found that 70% of women and 40% of men experience body dissatisfaction at some point in their lives. Negative body image doesn't reflect reality- it reflects perception.

2. The Impact of Negative Body Image

Negative body image can lead to:

- Emotional eating as a coping mechanism.

- Avoidance of healthy habits due to feelings of unworthiness.

- A constant cycle of dieting and bingeing caused by unrealistic goals.

Someone who feels ashamed of their body might avoid the gym, fearing judgment, which perpetuates inactivity and dissatisfaction.

3. How Body Positivity and Neutrality Help

You don't have to love every part of your body right away to improve your body image. Shifting toward *body neutrality*—acknowledging your body as a functional vessel—can help.

• **Body Positivity**: Celebrating your body regardless of size or shape.

• **Body Neutrality**: Focusing on what your body can do rather than how it looks.

Instead of fixating on the size of your thighs, appreciate that they allow you to walk, dance, or play with your kids.

Practical Strategies for Immediate Use

1. Challenge Negative Self-Talk

• Replace criticisms like *"I hate my stomach"* with neutral statements: *"My stomach carries me through the day."* Progress to positive affirmations like, *"I'm proud of how I'm working to improve my health."*

2. Curate Your Media Environment

• Unfollow social media accounts that promote unrealistic beauty standards. Follow people who inspire self-acceptance and celebrate diverse body types.

3. Practice Gratitude for Your Body

• Each day, write down three things your body does for you (e.g., "It allows me to hug my loved ones" or "It helps me enjoy nature"). Gratitude shifts focus from appearance to function.

4. Dress for Confidence Now

• Stop waiting until you've lost weight to wear clothes you love. Invest in outfits that make you feel good today.

5. Focus on Small Wins

• Celebrate non-scale victories like improved energy levels, better sleep, or completing a workout. These wins highlight progress beyond appearance.

Simplifying the Ideas

1.   **The Funhouse Mirror**
Negative body image is like looking at yourself in a distorted funhouse mirror. It doesn't reflect the truth but warps your perception. Rewiring your mindset is like stepping away from that mirror and seeing your true self.

2.   **Your Body as a Car**

Imagine your body as a car. It doesn't need to look like a sports car to function well. What matters is that it's reliable, well-maintained, and gets you where you need to go.

3.   **The Garden of Self-Acceptance**

Changing your body image is like tending a garden. You need to pull out the weeds of negative self-talk, plant seeds of gratitude, and nurture them daily to see growth over time.

Key Takeaways

• **Body image reflects perception, not reality**: Shift from criticism to gratitude.

• **Neutrality is a powerful tool**: Appreciate your body for its functions, not just its appearance.

• **Small changes create big results**: Challenge negative self-talk, focus on wins, and celebrate your progress.

Next Chapter: Building Habits That Stick

Rewiring your body image lays the foundation for long-term success. In the next chapter, we'll explore how to create habits that support your weight loss goals and make them stick for life.

This chapter motivates readers to view their bodies through a lens of compassion and practicality, empowering them to cultivate a healthier mindset while pursuing their goals.

Chapter 5: The Science of Habits & Weight Loss

Introduction: Small Changes, Big Results

Imagine if your daily actions effortlessly supported your weight loss goals. No more relying on fleeting motivation or willpower. Instead, habits—those automatic routines we don't think twice about—could carry you toward success.

The truth is, your habits shape your life. In this chapter, you'll learn how to create habits that align with your weight loss journey, sustain them long-term, and transform your lifestyle one step at a time.

Understanding Habits and How They Work

1. The Habit Loop

All habits follow the same cycle: **cue, routine, reward**.

- **Cue**: The trigger that starts the habit (e.g., feeling stressed).

- **Routine**: The action you take (e.g., eating a snack).

- **Reward**: The benefit you gain (e.g., feeling comforted).

To build new habits, you need to insert healthier routines into this cycle while keeping the cues and rewards intact.

Instead of reaching for cookies when stressed, replace the routine with taking a 5-minute walk, while the reward remains stress relief.

2. Why Motivation Isn't Enough
Motivation is great for starting, but it's unreliable in the long run. Habits, on the other hand, thrive on consistency, not inspiration.

Studies show it takes an average of **66 days** to form a new habit, depending on the complexity of the behaviour. Brushing your teeth is a habit you don't think about, not because you're motivated, but because it's ingrained in your routine.

3. The Power of Tiny Changes
Drastic lifestyle overhauls often fail because they're overwhelming. Small, incremental changes are more sustainable and easier to integrate into daily life. Start with a single habit, like drinking a glass of water before every meal, instead of attempting to overhaul your entire diet at once.

Practical Strategies for Immediate Use

1. Start Small

Focus on one habit at a time. For example:

- Add a daily 10-minute walk.

- Replace one sugary drink with water.

2. Pair Habits with Existing Routines *(Habit Stacking)*

Link a new habit to something you already do daily. For instance:

- After brushing your teeth, do 10 squats.

- While brewing your morning coffee, prepare a healthy snack for the day.

3. Use Visual Reminders

Set cues in your environment to remind you of your habits:

- Leave workout clothes by your bed as a cue to exercise in the morning.

- Keep a water bottle on your desk to encourage hydration.

4. Track Your Progress

- Use a habit tracker or journal to monitor consistency. Seeing your streak grow can motivate you to keep going.

5. Celebrate Small Wins

Reward yourself for sticking to habits, but avoid food-based rewards. Try:

- Treating yourself to a new book or workout gear.

- Celebrating with a relaxing activity.

Simplifying the Ideas

1. **The Snowball Effect**
Building habits is like rolling a snowball downhill. At first, it's small and takes effort to push, but as it gains momentum, it grows larger and rolls on its own.

2. **Planting Seeds**
Habits are like seeds: small and seemingly insignificant at first, but with consistent watering (effort), they grow into something impactful over time.

3. **The Brick Wall**
Each habit you build is like laying a brick. Alone, one brick may seem trivial, but over time, they form a sturdy wall—a foundation for your success.

Key Takeaways

- **Habits follow a loop**: Understand cues, routines, and rewards to change or build habits.

- **Start small and stack habits**: Pair new habits with existing ones for seamless integration.

- **Consistency beats motivation**: Focus on showing up, even if it's a small effort.

- **Celebrate progress**: Recognize wins to reinforce positive behaviour.

Next Chapter: Managing Stress Without Derailing Your Goals

Now that you've learned how to build lasting habits, we'll tackle one of the biggest obstacles to consistency: stress. In the next chapter, we'll explore effective stress management techniques that help you stay on track without turning to food.

This chapter provides actionable advice while empowering readers to embrace habit formation as a powerful tool for sustainable weight loss.
The Role of Stress and Sleep in Weight Loss

Chapter 6: Managing Stress Without Derailing Your Goals

Introduction: Taming the Stress Monster

Stress is one of the most significant roadblocks on a weight loss journey. Imagine this: you've had a rough day, and suddenly, the bag of chips on your counter starts calling your name. Before you know it, you've eaten through your feelings and derailed your progress.

Stress doesn't just impact your mood; it affects your body's ability to lose weight by increasing cortisol levels, which can trigger cravings for unhealthy foods and lead to emotional eating. This chapter will teach you how to recognize stress triggers, manage them effectively, and stay on track without relying on food for comfort.

The Relationship Between Stress and Weight Loss

1. Stress, Cortisol, and Cravings
When you're stressed, your body releases cortisol, a hormone that increases appetite and drives cravings for high-fat, sugary foods. This response is rooted in survival mechanisms from ancient times, but in today's world, it can sabotage your weight loss goals.

Research shows that 44% of adults eat more during stressful periods, often choosing calorie-dense comfort foods. Someone facing a tight deadline at work might grab a chocolate bar instead of a healthy snack because it provides quick, albeit temporary, relief.

2. Emotional Eating as a Coping Mechanism
Food is a common way to soothe stress because it provides a dopamine release, temporarily making you feel better. However, this creates a cycle: stress → eating → guilt → more stress. A person feeling lonely might turn to ice cream for comfort, but afterward, they feel guilty for overeating, compounding their stress.

3. The Long-Term Effects of Stress
Chronic stress not only hinders weight loss but can lead to:

- Fat storage, particularly in the abdominal area.

- Reduced motivation to exercise.

- Disrupted sleep, which further impacts metabolism and hunger hormones.

Practical Strategies for Immediate Use

1. Identify Your Stress Triggers

- Keep a journal to track what situations or emotions lead to stress eating. Awareness is the first step to breaking the cycle.

2. Replace Food with Non-Food Coping Mechanisms

- Instead of turning to snacks, try activities like:

- Going for a walk or run.

- Practicing deep breathing or meditation.

- Engaging in a creative hobby like drawing or knitting.

3. Build a Stress Management Toolkit

- Prepare in advance for high-stress situations. Examples include:

- Keeping a playlist of calming music.

- Setting up a "comfort box" with non-food items like a favorite book, journal, or essential oils.

4. Practice Mindful Eating

- Before eating, ask yourself: *Am I actually hungry, or am I stressed?* If it's stress, address the emotion first.

5. Get Active

- Exercise is one of the best stress relievers. It reduces cortisol and releases endorphins, improving both mood and motivation. Even a 10-minute walk can make a difference.

6. Use Positive Self-Talk

- Stress can amplify negative self-perceptions. Counteract this by affirming your progress and reminding yourself of your goals.

Analogies: Simplifying the Ideas

1. **The Pressure Cooker**
Think of stress as steam building up in a pressure cooker. If you don't release the steam regularly, the cooker explodes. Stress management techniques act as release valves, keeping you in control.

2. **The Quick Sand Trap**
Emotional eating is like stepping into quicksand. The more you struggle against stress by turning to food, the deeper you sink. Learning healthier coping mechanisms is your lifeline out.

3. **The Weather System**
Stress is like a storm: it can cloud your judgment and disrupt your plans, but it always passes. Building resilience is like carrying an umbrella—it doesn't stop the storm, but it helps you weather it.

Key Takeaways

- **Stress impacts weight loss directly**: Elevated cortisol levels increase cravings and fat storage.

- **Emotional eating creates a cycle**: Recognizing triggers is key to breaking it.

- **Healthier coping mechanisms reduce dependency on food**: Exercise, mindfulness, and self-care are effective alternatives.

Next Chapter: Cultivating Resilience and Consistency

Now that you've learned to manage stress, it's time to explore how resilience keeps you moving forward, even when life gets tough. In the next chapter, we'll focus on building consistency and staying motivated throughout your weight loss journey.

This chapter equips readers with actionable strategies to handle stress without derailing their progress, emphasizing mindfulness, self-awareness, and healthier coping mechanisms.

Chapter 7: Cultivating Resilience and Consistency

Introduction: Staying Strong When the Going Gets Tough

Weight loss isn't a straight road—it's a winding path full of unexpected detours and obstacles. Success isn't about never facing challenges; it's about bouncing back when you do. Resilience is the ability to recover from setbacks, while consistency is the art of showing up day after day, even when motivation wanes.

This chapter will teach you how to build the mental toughness and steady habits needed to navigate life's challenges without losing sight of your goals.

Building Resilience and Maintaining Consistency

1. What Is Resilience and Why Does It Matter?
Resilience is the mental strength to persevere through difficulties, adapt to change, and recover from setbacks. In weight loss, resilience helps you stay on track after a slip-up instead of spiraling into guilt or abandoning your goals altogether.

A resilient person who overeats at a party might acknowledge the misstep and return to their plan the next day, rather than letting one event derail their progress.

A 2020 study found that individuals with higher resilience are more likely to achieve long-term weight management success because they view setbacks as temporary, not defining.

2. The Myth of Perfection
Many people approach weight loss with an all-or-nothing mindset. However, perfection is unattainable, and striving for it often leads to burnout or giving up after one mistake.

    • **Key Point**: Consistency beats perfection. Small, sustained efforts are more effective than short bursts of extreme discipline. Walking 20 minutes a day may seem modest, but over a month, it adds up to 10 hours of activity—a meaningful impact.

3. The Role of Habits in Consistency
Consistency is built on habits, not motivation. By automating positive behaviors, you reduce the mental effort needed to stick to your plan. Research shows that consistent adherence to small changes, like tracking food intake or maintaining a sleep schedule, is the most reliable predictor of weight loss success.

Practical Strategies for Immediate Use

1. Reframe Setbacks as Learning Opportunities

    • Instead of thinking, *"I failed,"* ask yourself, *"What can I learn from this?"* For example:

    • If you skipped a workout because you were tired, evaluate whether you're getting enough sleep or scheduling exercise at the right time.

2. Use the 80/20 Rule

- Focus on being consistent 80% of the time, allowing flexibility for life's ups and downs. This approach reduces guilt and keeps you on track long-term.

3. Celebrate Small Wins

- Recognize daily successes to maintain motivation. Examples:

- Preparing a healthy meal instead of ordering takeout.

- Drinking an extra glass of water during the day.

4. Plan for Challenges

- Anticipate potential obstacles and create a plan:

- If travelling, pack healthy snacks or identify restaurants with balanced options.

- If facing a busy week, schedule shorter workouts instead of skipping them altogether.

5. Surround Yourself with Support

- Share your goals with a friend, join a community, or seek an accountability partner. External encouragement can boost resilience and consistency.

Simplifying the Ideas

1. **The Rubber Band Effect**
Resilience is like a rubber band. It stretches under pressure but doesn't snap. Even after setbacks, it returns to its original form, just like you can bounce back after challenges.

2. **Brick by Brick**
Consistency is like building a wall, one brick at a time. Each small action—choosing a healthy snack, completing a workout—adds to the structure. Even if one brick is misplaced, the wall remains intact if you keep building.

3. **The Tortoise and the Hare**
Remember the classic fable: slow and steady wins the race. Consistency (the tortoise) will always outpace bursts of effort (the hare) in the long run.

Key Takeaways

- **Resilience allows you to bounce back**: Setbacks are temporary and offer opportunities for growth.

• **Consistency, not perfection, drives success**: Focus on sustainable, small actions rather than flawless execution.

• **Build habits and plan for challenges**: Automate positive behaviors and create strategies for when life gets tough.

Next Chapter: The Power of Self-Compassion in Weight Loss

Now that you've built resilience and consistency, it's time to address a critical mindset shift: practicing self-compassion. In the next chapter, you'll learn how to be kinder to yourself, which is essential for staying motivated and achieving lasting change.

This chapter encourages readers to view their journey as a process, equipping them with tools to persevere through setbacks while focusing on consistent, manageable progress.

Chapter 8: The Power of Self-Compassion in Weight Loss

Introduction: Be Your Own Best Friend

If you want to achieve long-term weight loss success, the most important relationship you'll need to nurture is the one with yourself. Too often, people beat themselves up over mistakes, missteps, or imperfections in their journey. They fall into the trap of self-criticism, which can lead to discouragement, burnout, and ultimately giving up on their goals.

Self-compassion is the antidote to this destructive pattern. It's about being kind and understanding toward yourself, especially when things don't go as planned. In this chapter, you'll learn how self-compassion can be a powerful tool in your weight loss journey, helping you stay motivated, resilient, and empowered—no matter what challenges arise.

Understanding Self-Compassion and Its Role in Weight Loss

1. What Is Self-Compassion?
Self-compassion is treating yourself with the same kindness and understanding that you would offer to a friend who is struggling. It involves three key components:

• **Self-kindness**: Being gentle with yourself when you fail or make mistakes.

• **Common humanity**: Recognizing that everyone faces struggles—you're not alone in your challenges.

- **Mindfulness**: Acknowledging your feelings without judgment, accepting that pain and discomfort are part of the human experience.

When you skip a workout, instead of harshly criticizing yourself, you acknowledge the slip-up and remind yourself that everyone misses a workout now and then. You then refocus on getting back on track.

2. Self-Criticism Hurts More Than It Helps

The more you criticize yourself, the more you're likely to give up on your goals. Studies show that self-criticism is linked to higher levels of stress and lower levels of motivation. This negative feedback loop only perpetuates feelings of failure and discouragement, making it harder to stay consistent.

Research published in the journal *Health Psychology* found that people who practiced self-compassion were more likely to engage in healthy behaviours like exercising and eating well, while those who were self-critical were more prone to emotional eating and bingeing.

3. The Impact of Self-Compassion on Long-Term Weight Loss

Self-compassion isn't just a nice-to-have trait; it's a critical component for long-term success. When you are kind to yourself, you're more likely to stay committed to your weight loss journey, even after setbacks. It helps reduce stress, promotes healthy decision-making, and encourages a mindset of growth rather than perfectionism.

A woman who struggles with emotional eating can practice self-compassion by recognizing her feelings of stress, offering herself comfort in non-food ways, and forgiving herself for past overeating, rather than using it as an excuse to give up.

Practical Strategies for Immediate Use

1. Practice Self-Kindness Daily

- When you make a mistake, remind yourself, *"I am doing my best. It's okay to have setbacks."*

- Instead of saying, *"I'm so weak,"* try, *"I'm human, and I can learn from this."*

2. Reframe Your Inner Dialogue

- Replace critical thoughts with positive affirmations.

- Instead of *"I can't stick to my plan,"* try, *"I am capable of making small improvements each day."*

3. Treat Yourself Like You Would a Friend

• If a friend were in your shoes, what would you say to them? Treat yourself with the same compassion and understanding.

• If a friend had a bad day and ate comfort food, you wouldn't scold them. Instead, you would encourage them to start fresh tomorrow. Do the same for yourself.

4. Embrace Imperfection

• Let go of the need for perfection. Progress is not linear, and everyone has ups and downs.

• Celebrate small victories, even if they don't seem monumental. Every step forward counts.

5. Practice Mindfulness

• Practice mindfulness exercises, such as deep breathing or body scans, to help you stay present and reduce judgmental thinking.

• Take a moment to pause and check in with how you're feeling before acting on a craving or emotional response.

Simplifying the Ideas

1. **The Garden Analogy**
Think of yourself as a garden. If a flower wilts, you don't yell at it or pull it up. You water it, give it sunshine, and allow it to grow. Similarly, when you make mistakes, treat yourself with the same care and patience you would give to a plant that needs nurturing.

2. **The Coach Analogy**
Imagine having a coach who is harsh and critical all the time versus a coach who is supportive, encouraging, and kind. Which coach would help you achieve your goals? Self-compassion is like being your own supportive coach, encouraging you to keep going, even when the journey gets tough.

3. **The Slippery Slope Analogy**
Criticizing yourself is like walking down a slippery slope—each negative thought makes it easier to slide further away from your goals. Self-compassion, on the other hand, is like having a firm grip that helps you regain balance and move forward with confidence.

Key Takeaways

• **Self-compassion is essential**: Treat yourself with kindness and understanding, especially when you slip up.

• **Self-criticism is counterproductive**: Negative self-talk leads to stress, emotional eating, and a lack of motivation.

• **Embrace imperfection**: Progress takes time, and every mistake is an opportunity to grow.

• **Be your own best friend**: Offer yourself the same support and encouragement you would give a loved one.

Next Chapter: Finding Your "Why" for Lasting Motivation

In the next chapter, we will dive into the importance of discovering your deeper motivations—your "why"—for losing weight. When you connect with your true purpose, you'll have a powerful, sustainable source of motivation that goes beyond just fitting into a pair of jeans.

This chapter focuses on the transformative power of self-compassion in weight loss, helping readers shift from self-criticism to self-encouragement, fostering a healthy, sustainable approach to their goals.

Chapter 9: Finding Your "Why" for Lasting Motivation

Introduction: Digging Deeper Than the Scale

It's easy to get motivated by external goals like losing 10 pounds or fitting into a smaller dress size, but these reasons often lack the staying power needed for long-term success. Motivation can be fleeting—what keeps you going day after day, especially when faced with obstacles, is something deeper.

In this chapter, we'll explore the power of discovering your true motivation—the deeper *why* that fuels your weight loss journey. When your motivation is rooted in a sense of purpose, it becomes the driving force that helps you overcome challenges, stay consistent, and create lasting change in your life.

Understanding the Power of Your "Why"

1. Motivation Beyond the Surface
Surface-level goals, like fitting into a specific clothing size, may inspire you initially, but they won't sustain you in the long run. True motivation comes from understanding why weight loss is meaningful to you beyond the physical appearance. When you identify your "why," you tap into a deeper emotional connection that strengthens your commitment.

Instead of focusing on fitting into a smaller dress, consider why that goal is important. Do you want more energy to keep up with your kids? Are you striving for better health so you can travel or live an active lifestyle?

Research from the American Psychological Association suggests that people who identify intrinsic motivations (like improved health or personal well-being) are more likely to succeed at maintaining weight loss over time than those focused solely on external rewards.

2. Connecting to Your Deeper Purpose

Your "why" is the emotional core of your weight loss journey. It's about identifying what you truly want to feel, achieve, or experience through your transformation. Connecting to this deeper purpose can help you stay focused on your goals, even when progress seems slow.

A person's "why" might be to improve their health so they can be there for their family, walk their daughter down the aisle, or live to see their grandchildren grow up. When challenges arise, that "why" becomes a powerful reminder of what's at stake.

3. Your "Why" Provides Consistency

When motivation wanes, your deeper purpose will serve as your anchor. While daily motivation may fluctuate, your "why" doesn't change—it stays constant and provides a sense of direction. It gives you a reason to push through difficult moments, helping you make choices that align with your long-term goals.

If you're tempted to skip a workout or eat something unhealthy, asking yourself, *"How does this choice support my purpose?"* can help you realign and stay on track.

Practical Strategies for Immediate Use

1. Write Down Your "Why"

Take time to reflect on what truly motivates you. Is it improving your health? Gaining more energy? Feeling confident in your skin? Write down your answers and keep them visible as a daily reminder.

2. Create a Vision Board

- Visualizing your goals makes them more tangible. Create a vision board with images or words that represent your deeper purpose—things that inspire you to stay committed.

3. Dig Deeper with the "5 Whys"

- When you identify a surface-level reason (e.g., "I want to lose weight"), ask yourself why that's important five times. Each answer will bring you closer to your true, underlying motivation.

- **Example:**

Why do you want to lose weight?

- *To feel more confident.*

  - *Why do you want to feel more confident?*

- *Because I want to go to social events without feeling self-conscious.*

  - *Why do you want to feel good at social events?*

- *Because I want to connect with people without fear of judgment.*

4. Revisit Your "Why" Regularly

- Your motivation may evolve as your journey progresses. Revisit your "why" regularly and adjust it as needed to keep it aligned with your goals.

5. Share Your "Why" with Others

- Tell a trusted friend or family member about your deeper motivations. Having someone to hold you accountable to your "why" can strengthen your resolve.

Simplifying the Ideas

1. **The Compass Analogy**
Think of your "why" as a compass. It guides you through the journey, ensuring you stay on course, even when the path gets difficult. Without a compass, you might wander aimlessly, but with a strong "why," you know exactly where you're headed.

2. **The Fuel Analogy**
Your "why" is the fuel for your journey. It's what keeps you going when the engine of motivation starts to run low. Without a strong source of fuel, your efforts will stall, but with a meaningful "why," you'll keep moving forward, no matter the obstacles.

3. **The Root of a Tree Analogy**
Your surface goals are like the leaves of a tree—important, but easily affected by the wind. Your "why" is the root—deep, strong, and unwavering, no matter how much the branches bend. By staying grounded in your "why," you ensure that your weight loss journey remains strong and sustainable.

Key Takeaways

- **Surface goals won't sustain you long-term**: True motivation comes from connecting to your deeper purpose.

• **Your "why" is your anchor**: It provides clarity and consistency, especially when motivation fluctuates.

• **Identify your "why" now**: Reflect on what truly drives you and revisit it regularly to stay aligned with your goals.

Next Chapter: Celebrating Progress and Building Long-Term Success

In the next chapter, we'll explore the importance of celebrating your progress, no matter how small. Acknowledging milestones, both big and small, is essential to sustaining your momentum and ensuring long-term success.

This chapter helps readers discover their deeper motivations, turning weight loss into a purpose-driven journey. By finding their "why," readers can stay committed, resilient, and focused on achieving their long-term health and wellness goals.

Chapter 10: Celebrating Progress and Building Long-Term Success

Introduction: The Power of Small Wins

In the pursuit of weight loss, it's easy to get caught up in the end goal—the final number on the scale, the ultimate transformation. However, focusing solely on the end result can undermine your success in the long run. The key to lasting change is in recognizing and celebrating the small victories along the way.

In this chapter, we will explore why celebrating progress is essential for maintaining motivation, boosting self-confidence, and building a foundation for long-term success. By acknowledging your wins—no matter how small—you shift your mindset from one of scarcity and frustration to one of abundance and achievement.

Why Celebrating Progress Fuels Long-Term Success

1. Progress Is Built on Consistency, Not Perfection
Many people expect perfection from themselves and feel defeated when they don't see immediate, dramatic results. However, lasting weight loss comes from small, consistent actions over time. Every healthy choice, every workout completed, every step forward is a piece of the puzzle.

If you focus only on the weight you've lost in a given week or month, you may overlook the habits you've built—like regularly eating balanced meals or exercising several times a week. These habits are the real markers of progress.

Research from the *Journal of Applied Behavioral Analysis* shows that individuals who celebrate their small victories are more likely to maintain behavior change and have better long-term success in health-related goals.

2. Celebrating Boosts Motivation and Reinforces Positive Behaviors
When you celebrate your wins, your brain releases dopamine, a neurotransmitter associated with pleasure and reward. This helps reinforce the positive behaviors that led to those successes, making it easier to continue those behaviors in the future.

After completing a challenging workout, celebrating with a healthy treat or taking a moment to acknowledge your achievement strengthens the desire to continue working out.

3. The Role of Self-Compassion in Celebration
Celebrating progress isn't just about acknowledging your victories—it's about being kind to yourself in the process. Often, people are more comfortable celebrating others than themselves. However, you deserve to celebrate your efforts and the hard work you've put in.

If you hit a milestone, like losing 5 pounds or running your first 5K, take a moment to honor that success. Give yourself permission to feel proud and acknowledge the dedication that got you there. This boosts self-esteem and creates a positive cycle of success.

Practical Strategies for Celebrating Progress

1. Keep a "Win Journal"

- Write down your daily or weekly wins, no matter how small they seem. This could be something as simple as saying "no" to an unhealthy snack or getting up early to exercise. By writing these down, you're actively training your brain to notice and celebrate your progress.

2. Set Micro-Goals and Reward Yourself

- Break down your larger weight loss goal into smaller, achievable milestones. For example, aim for a goal of walking 10,000 steps per day for a week. Once you hit your goal, reward yourself with something that aligns with your values—maybe a relaxing bath or a new workout outfit.

3. Share Your Successes with Others

- Tell a friend, family member, or social media community about your progress. Sharing your wins with others increases accountability and allows others to celebrate with you, creating a positive feedback loop of motivation.

4. Create Non-Food Rewards

• Often, food rewards can undo the progress you've made. Instead, choose rewards that support your weight loss goals—like a massage, a new book, or a day out doing something active that you enjoy.

5. Reflect on Your Journey Regularly

• Take time at the end of each week or month to reflect on how far you've come. Look back at where you started, what challenges you've overcome, and how you've grown. This reflection not only helps you recognize your progress but also reinforces your commitment to the process.

Simplifying the Concepts

1.   **The Brick Wall Analogy**
Building long-term success is like constructing a brick wall. Every small achievement—whether it's losing a pound, completing a workout, or resisting a craving—is a brick in the wall. If you focus solely on the finished wall (the end result), you might get discouraged. But by recognizing each brick, you appreciate the progress you're making in real-time.

2.   **The Garden Analogy**
Weight loss is like growing a garden. You don't plant a seed today and expect to see a fully grown tree tomorrow. You water, nurture, and take care of it every day. By celebrating the small sprouts that begin to emerge—whether it's increased energy, improved mood, or even a small loss in inches—you're building a flourishing garden that will eventually bear fruit.

3.   **The Marathon Analogy**
Weight loss is a marathon, not a sprint. Just like a marathon runner doesn't wait until they've crossed the finish line to celebrate their progress, you shouldn't wait until your ultimate goal is reached. Celebrate every mile marker—the small victories—because each step brings you closer to your destination.

Key Takeaways

• **Focus on consistency, not perfection**: Progress is built from small, sustainable actions.

• **Celebrate every win**: Acknowledge your achievements, both big and small, to reinforce positive behaviors and maintain motivation.

• **Self-compassion is key**: Be kind to yourself in the process and allow yourself to feel proud of your efforts.

• **Reward yourself thoughtfully**: Choose rewards that support your goals and help you stay on track.

Conclusion: Embracing the Journey

As you come to the end of this book, it's important to reflect on how far you've come—not just in your understanding of weight loss but in shifting the way you view yourself and your journey. True success in weight management is not measured by a number on the scale but by the resilience, self-awareness, and habits you've cultivated along the way.

We began this journey by uncovering the hidden forces that influence weight loss—the beliefs, emotions, and habits that often go unnoticed yet hold immense power. By addressing these psychological factors, you've unlocked a deeper understanding of what drives your behaviors and how to rewrite the narratives that no longer serve you.

This process is not about perfection but about progress. Setbacks are not failures; they are opportunities to learn, grow, and adapt. Every step, no matter how small, contributes to the greater picture of your health and well-being. By embracing this mindset, you free yourself from the all-or-nothing thinking that often derails progress and instead develop a lifetime mindset of growth and balance.

Your journey is deeply personal, and your success will be defined by how well you align your habits with your values and goals. Remember, sustainable change takes time, patience, and self-compassion. Celebrate the milestones you achieve along the way, and remember to honor your body and mind for the effort and progress they make every day.

What's Next?

Your work doesn't end here. The insights and tools you've gained from this book are meant to be practiced and adapted as you grow. Life will continue to bring challenges, but now you have the mindset and strategies to navigate them with confidence. Consider the following steps to deepen your transformation:

- **Journaling**: Use the exercises in this book to continue exploring your thoughts, behaviors, and goals.
- **Community**: Surround yourself with a support system that uplifts and encourages you.
- **Accountability**: Regularly revisit the goals and habits you've set to ensure they align with your evolving lifestyle.

Your Call to Action

The most powerful tool you possess is your ability to choose. Choose to approach each day with curiosity and kindness toward yourself. Choose to view obstacles as stepping stones. And most importantly, choose to believe that you are capable of achieving lasting change.

Weight loss is no longer just about "losing weight." It's about gaining confidence, clarity, and control over your life. As you continue your journey, remember: *The only limits are the ones you place on yourself. Rewrite your story, one choice at a time, starting today.*

Here's to your lifelong success and the healthy, empowered future you deserve!